Juicing:

Your Liquid Nutritional Supplement

Deborah Lee

Woodland Publishing
Pleasant Grove, Utah

Woodland Publishing
P.O. Box 160
Pleasant Grove, UT
84062

Table of Contents

Woodland Publishing
P.O. Box 160
Pleasant Grove, UT
84062

Juicing

Introduction

The human body is a marvelous machine. When given the proper tools, it has the ability to repair and regenerate itself when injuries and illnesses develop. All cells, tissues, and organs work in harmony, quietly and without fanfare. They don't shout for approval and say, "Look at what we are doing for you." However, when they need attention, they certainly let us know through pain, fatigue, and other manifestations. Usually, people don't think about the importance of health until it diminishes or is gone. Then they try to find ways to restore that vitality they had taken for granted. On the other hand, if we employ preventive maintenance in the first place, we can live long, happy and healthy lives.

You are probably wondering where juicing fits into the healthy scheme of things. You are also probably wondering what it can do for you. Juicing can be viewed as a natural health supplement; it is an adjunct to a nutritious diet. In addition to improving your diet, juicing can be restorative and regenerative to those who have imbalances in their health and are experiencing illness and discomfort. Juicing's main strength is that it cleanses and flushes toxins from the cells so they can function properly, thus helping to maintain optimal health.

Moreover, those who are ill can tolerate juices where it may be difficult to chew and digest an entire fruit or vegetable. Raw juices only take approximately 15 minutes to digest. You can receive instant nutrition for very little energy expenditure. This is especially important when you are ill, and your body cannot afford to expend a large amount of energy. The vitamins, minerals, and enzymes are immediately absorbed into the circulatory system and transferred into the cells of the body where they are used to promote health and vitality.

Raw juices also promote an alkaline balance in the body. Famous nutrition expert Dr. Bernard Jensen explains:

> There has been much talk in the last few years about acid and alkaline foods. It has been determined that for optimum health, a body should be slightly alkaline. If the body becomes too acid or too alkaline, illness and disease will result.
>
> When we speak of an acid body, we need to understand the notion of pH, or relative acidity-alkalinity, in the standard terminology of chemistry. The pH scale is from 1 to 14, with 7 representing neutrality, neither acid nor alkaline. Most living things require an acid-alkaline environment of between pH 5.5 and 8 to survive. Outside of this range, they sicken and die.

> When we use an excessively acid diet (meat and potatoes every day, for example), large quantities of sodium, potassium, calcium, magnesium, and other acid-neutralizing chemicals are constantly used up in preventing tissue damage. The problem is, these chemical elements are drawn from the tissues and must be replaced, or deficiencies will occur, soon followed by disease symptoms. Over alkaline diets are seldom found, but they would also be harmful over the long term.
>
> For these reasons, my food laws say we must have six vegetables and two fruits each day, which make up the 80 percent of the alkaline-forming foods required, and one starch and one protein, the 20 percent acid-forming foods required.[1]

Raw vegetable and fruit juices contain mega-nutrients. When you consider that it takes five to eight averaged-size carrots to make one 8-10 ounce glass of juice, you know that glass of juice is brimming with beta carotene, calcium, enzymes and other goodies naturally found in the carrot. The best part about it is that all nutrients are provided in the ratios and spectrums that nature intended. The body utilizes foods in their natural state much better than it does when that food has been manipulated, refined, or altered in any way. The body recognizes it immediately as having great value and literally pulls the nutrients into the cells. It is a true scientific and biological fact that "you are not what you eat; you are what you absorb." You could take a million vitamin pills and if your body did not assimilate the nutrients effectively, you would receive no benefit from taking them.

Naturally Colored Nutrients

What is more refreshing than a glass of pure juice with all of its native goodness? The deep hues of various fruits and vegetables are not only appealing to the eye, they are also sources of powerful phyto (plant) nutrients. Nature supplies an abundant rainbow of natural pigments that provide a feast for the eyes and the immune system. Take grapes, for instance. The purple and red skins of this fruit, as well as cherries and members of the blueberry family, burst with antioxidants known as "proanthocyanidins." Antioxidants help prevent damage to cells from unstable molecules known as free radicals. Free radicals are generated both inside and outside the body. Free radicals are by-products of normal processes of digestion and metabolism. Exercise can promote free radical production. In addition, external factors such as air pollution, overheated cooking oils, and charred meats from barbequing and grilling can introduce free radicals into the body. Free radicals can attack healthy cells and turn them into sick cells. The primary culprits responsible for premature aging and different types of sicknesses, free radicals are not agents to be disregarded. Fresh fruits and vegetables, with their abundant antioxidant nutrients, are an inexpensive but potent guard against free radical damage.

The green color of cruciferous vegetable family members, such as broccoli, cabbage, and kale, offers compounds called "indoles" that reduce the risk of breast cancer by inactivating certain harmful estrogens.

The ruddy hues of tomatoes, pink grapefruit, and watermelon contain appreciable amounts of vitamin C, as well as a substance known as lycopene—a cancer-preventing antioxidant.

Carrots, cantaloupe, apricots, papaya, and other orange-pigmented fruits and vegetables are rich in a particular carotenoid called beta carotene. Research shows that this antioxidant vitamin, which the body can convert to vitamin A, is a dynamic weapon against cancer. Carotene also promotes the body's production of "visual purple" or rhodopdsin, which helps prevent night blindness. Leafy greens are also powerhouses of beta carotene, as well as chlorophyll, a substance that can bind to cancer-causing chemicals in the intestinal tract and inhibit their absorption by the body.

As you can see, there is more than meets the eye in the tantalizing array of colors in nature's palette.

The Importance of Enzymes

What helps nutrients get to the cells, tissues and organs? The catalysts or "helpers" are the enzymes found naturally in raw foods. Cooked foods do not contain live enzymes. The enzymes that were originally there were killed when the food was heated.

Health author Humbart Santillo explains:

> An "enzyme" is said to be a protein molecule and each acts in a certain way in the body doing specific jobs such as digesting food, building protein in the bones and skin and aiding detoxification, to name a few.
>
> Once we cook food at high temperatures, however, the

enzyme is destroyed. It no longer carries on its designated function. Although the physical protein molecule is still present, it has lost its life force. Much like a battery that has lost its power, the physical structure remains; but the electrical energy which once animated it is no longer present.

An enzyme is the invisible activity or energy factor and not just the protein molecule itself. So, for clarity, let us agree that a protein molecule is a carrier of the enzyme activity, much like the light bulb is the carrier for an electrical current."[2]

The Importance of Fresh Juices

Why not drink the juices from the grocery store? Fresh juices can flush the system of toxins. However, canned or bottled juices cannot do this, for their enzymes are dead. These products are sterile. The nutrients, for the most part, are destroyed. In order to can or bottle commercial juices, the juice must be heated to at least 175 degrees Fahrenheit for several minutes to preserve it for transportation and storage. At 130 degrees, the enzymes are totally destroyed. The digestive organs, (especially the pancreas), are then burdened because they have to work extra hard to provide enzymes that the foods or juices are lacking for the body to utilize any part of them. When the digestive system is weakened, other parts of the body are affected, and one thing leads to another until disease takes over.

The renowned Dr. John R. Christopher, N.D., M.H., explained the above information this way:

One of the finest ways to obtain necessary nutrients in the diet is through the intake of raw fruit and vegetable juices. Many of the readily available vitamins and minerals in fruits and vegetables are needlessly lost during cooking, boiling, frying and other ruinous food preparation processes. Nature presents fruits and vegetables to us in a wholesome state, containing all the essentials which can sustain a high quality of life in a healthy body. Man, in his insatiable desire to improve upon nature, usually creates a product that hardly resembles the natural design in appearance or function.

We see the market shelves (and this includes the health food stores) loaded with all sorts of 'health-giving,' bottled juices derived from numerous sources—this includes the common garden variety vegetables and the most exotic tropically grown fruits. The main thing these juices have in common is this: THEY ARE ALL DEAD. During the bottling or canning process the precious juices are heated to temperatures far above the sun's ripening rays in the field or orchard. We know that whenever a food is heated above approximately 130 degrees Fahrenheit, many of the life-giving enzymes are destroyed. The vitamins and minerals contained within the substance are converted to inorganic and unassimilable toxins. These inorganic poisons are extremely detrimental to the system because often they cannot be easily eliminated by weakened organs.[3]

The Process of Digestion

The process of digestion begins in the mouth. The saliva mixes with food and breaks carbohydrates into sugars, thus "pre-digesting" them. The enzyme ptyalin is responsible for this job. Even juices need to go through this step. Since you cannot "chew" juices, swish the first two or three swallows of juice around in your mouth and let it mix with your saliva thoroughly before ingesting. This will prepare the juices for better assimilation by the body. Dr. John R. Christopher explains it this way:

> With fresh juice taken within a few minutes after squeezing, the vital source of energy goes directly into the bloodstream. All juices should be sipped slowly and 'chewed' like solid food. They should be swished around in the mouth and thoroughly mixed in the saliva in order to properly begin the digestive process. Many juices are rich and not compatible with the gastric juices when an insufficient amount of saliva is present. This may result in discomfort or regurgitation. So juices should not be gulped or drunk quickly in large amounts.[4]

Juices, just as any other food source, need to be digested in order to be effectively assimilated by the body.

It takes more energy from the body to digest food than for any other bodily process. This is particularly true of meats and heavy starches. This is why a person can feel very sleepy or tired after consuming a meal of these concentrated foods. The body is using all of its energy to process the food. Meat itself takes six to eight hours to digest. Contrast this with fresh, raw juices. The body immediately takes in the nutrition, without having to break down. Juicing gives our digestive tract a rest, a vacation, so to speak.

The Importance of Detoxification

Everyone has toxins or poisons that accumulate in the body over the years. This is a consequence of existence. If you eat, breathe, and drink, you get them. Toxins come from airborne pollutants, preservatives in foods, parasites in water and meats; the sources are many. The older we get, the more toxins we build up. However, depending on lifestyle, some people accumulate more toxins than others do. As time passes, the body has a harder and harder time of eliminating these burdens, and the liver (the primary detoxifying organ of the body) becomes weary and weak. The poisons interfere with health because the intestinal tract and blood stream are affected, and the end result is a weakened immune system. This interference causes a "biochemical imbalance" because proper cell function is disrupted. The thought processes and emotions can be affected, as well as physical well-being. People who chronically experience anxiety, depression, hostility, fear, and the inability to fall asleep may not be properly nourished. Dr. Ann Wigmore explains:

> In order to permanently eliminate a condition, we must first work to dissolve the cause. Our mental thought patterns can actually create a disease where there was none before. Also, where there actually is a disease, if we continually think about it, the disease will tend to not

> improve, or it might even get worse. Other thought patterns which contribute to the negative side of health are CRITICISM, ANGER and RESENTMENT. For instance, criticism indulged in long enough will often lead to diseases such as arthritis. Resentment long-held festers in the body to eventually even lead to tumors and cancer."

Dr. Wigmore has long advocated the virtues of green juices, especially wheat grass juice. She states:

> When warnings start to manifest, such as pain, swelling, fever, cold, weakness, tiredness—our bodies tell us we are unhealthy and a change must be made. Our bodies are no longer able to handle the lifestyle and food that is being delivered to the cells. If the cells are not being nourished properly, and are over-burdened with waste from unused food, sickness is the result. Or, if we repress these warnings in any way, then the body develops even a more serious health condition. Then these conditions degenerate even further, manifesting through diseases such as arthritis, heart conditions, high blood pressure, asthma, premature aging, and cancer, as well as the diseases which affect the nerves such as multiple sclerosis, lupus, and epilepsy. . . . As stated before, in order to avoid any health problems, we must give the body live food nourishment so that the cells can do their cleansing and rebuilding, thereby keeping us happy.[5]

As the body throws off poisons that may have been stored for many years, flu-like symptoms may result. These annoyances will eventually disappear as the body is cleansed, and you will experience greater energy levels.

Many cases of stubborn obesity can be resolved as the body releases toxins. A sluggish metabolism can be restored to normal as the intestinal tract is cleansed and the body is able to accept more nutrition through the intestinal walls. In doing so, it will naturally balance bodily processes — including the metabolism. As an added benefit, cravings for high-calorie foods and snacks will disappear as the body is satisfied with the mega-nutrients supplied through natural, raw juices.

Why does some people's skin turn orange when they drink a lot of carrot juice? Does the pigment in the carrots turn the skin that color? Dr. N.W. Walker explains:

> It is ignorance of the functions of the body that would make anyone believe such nonsense. It is just as absurd to expect the color pigment of the carrot to come through the skin as to expect the red of the beet or green of the spinach to come through. Whenever, after drinking juices, yellow or brown appears though the skin, it is an indication that the liver is eliminating stale bile and other waste matter in greater quantities than the eliminative organs can handle so that some of the elimination takes place through the pores of the skin, which is perfectly normal. If the body is toxic, such also may be the case. When we continue to drink vegetable juices, however, the discoloration eventually disappears.[6]

Periodic cleansing and then maintaining a high level of nutrition through diet are keys to optimal health. With the necessary nutrients, your body will be able to repair cells, tissues, and organs and keep them functioning at their peak. You will have exceptional energy; you will experience emotional stability and calmness, and you will not have to wait until an illness forces a cleanse upon you. Actually, the body will cleanse on its own when the toxins become too high and needs to rid itself of debris. A cold is nothing more than a cleanse. A virus is just the "catalyst" to initiate the cleanse. A lot of people come in contact with cold viruses but do not get sick. If a virus has nothing to work with, it cannot penetrate healthy, strong cells and membranes. Many natural health care practitioners believe that viruses or bacteria cannot initiate a cleanse and trigger the body to release mucus if the system is clean.

If you are missing a balanced ratio of vitamins and minerals in the body, energy synthesis will not take place in the body. You will feel tired and run-down. Cleansing and rebuilding are the keys to regaining health.

Balancing Body Chemistry

Proper mineral and vitamin ratios are essential for the body's engine to run smoothly and well. These two classifications of nutrients are interdependent; that is, they rely on one another to perform their roles. This process is also known as "synergism." If nutrients are not working in synchronization, biochemical imbalances may result. As a consequence, many physical and emotional ailments can emerge. Disruption of internal biochemical harmony can manifest itself as anxiety, fear, hostility, depression, insomnia, and a host of other seemingly unrelated symptoms.

Poor digestion, constipation, low energy levels, and other abnormal physical conditions can also come from biochemical imbalances. If one nutrient is out of balance, it can cause a chain reaction of other problems. Nature supplies vitamins, minerals, enzymes, and other vital substances in fruits and vegetables in their proper and balanced quantities.

When a person is sick, the body naturally conserves energy to try and heal. The appetite is decreased, to free up the energy needed to rebuild. At this time the body cannot adequately assimilate food. Food can act as a poison at this time because the body will not be able to properly break it down. Juice fasting is the answer. It is the way to get healing nutrients into the system, while reserving the energy needed for digestion. Fasting (going without food) does not give the body the materials it needs to rebuild and heal. Because fruit juices are considered the cleansers of the body and vegetable juices the builders (because of the high mineral content), it is suggested that fruit juices be taken in the morning and vegetable juices in the afternoon and evening.

The glands are the organs of the body responsible for essential functions and procedures that keep the body machinery going. Endocrine glands secrete minute amounts of substances known as hormones. A hormone is "a complex chemical substance produced in one part or organ of the body that initiates or regulates the activity of an organ or a group of cells in another part of the body."[7] In order to do their job, glands must have a proper ratio of minerals. The body cannot manufacture minerals, but is entirely dependent upon dietary sources. Today's modern farming methods have depleted the nation's topsoils of vital nutrients. The plants grown on these soils, consequently cannot draw from that which is not there, so they, too, are deficient and of inferior quality. Actually, the soils have been deficient for a long time. Consider this information that was published in the

June 1936 issue of *Cosmopolitan Magazine.* Dr. Charles Northern was quoted as saying:

> Do you know that most of us today are suffering from certain dangerous diet deficiencies which cannot be remedied until the depleted soils from which our foods come are brought into proper mineral balance? The alarming fact is that foods—fruits and vegetables and grains—now being raised on millions of acres of land that no longer contain enough of certain needed minerals, are starving us—no matter how much of them we eat!

Organically Grown Produce Sources Are Best

If possible, make your juices from vegetables that have been grown on organic, composted soils. In addition, commercial farming methods employ toxic herbicides and insecticides as part of the growing and harvesting process. These remain in the fibers and skins of the vegetables. It is common knowledge that herbicides and pesticides are very dangerous and can cause cancer. Therefore, unless you use organically grown vegetables, do not retain the leftover roughage pulp to add nutrition to other dishes, as some people do who do not want to waste that part of the food.

If you can get it, organically grown produce is best for juicing or for just eating. However, according to N. W. Walker, one of the world's top authorities on juicing, the fiber is where the toxins accumulate. He explains:

There is a little-known fact regarding the effect of pesticides on our vegetables and fruits, which should be given much publicity in these times.

We have been able to determine that pesticides and sprays may be injurious in the consumption of vegetables and fruits, it is the FIBERS of such foods that collect these toxins. The enzymes, atoms, and molecules are allergic to them.

Furthermore, under the very best soil conditions the use of sprays and pesticides will enter into the plants and roots but will be completely absorbed by the fibers of the plants and roots. The plants will continue to grow and thrive, not because of these toxins, but in spite of them. Why? Because the enzymes, atoms, and molecules will continue to carry on their work without the interruption in spite of the poison-saturated fibers.

The question arises: How to get the enzymes, atoms and molecules from our vegetables without using the poisoned fibers? After all, these enzymes, atoms and molecules are the nourishing elements we require. The fibers have virtually no nourishing value.

The answer is simple: by the process of triturating the vegetables, the cells of the fibers are split open and these elements are released. The result is a pulp almost as fine as apple butter. These elements are just as allergic to toxins as oil is to water. Therefore, they will retain their virgin virtue by not mixing integrally with the triturated fibers.

By squeezing this triturated pulp through proper straining material, the juice containing enzymes, atoms and molecules is extracted from the fibers and the toxins with which they are saturated.

. . . However, our use of the electric triturator and hydraulic press does not rule out the use of centrifugal machines. While it is recognized that by centrifugal action we cannot extract ALL of the enzymes, atoms and molecules; nevertheless, the use of a filter in the centrifugal extractor prevents the fibers from mixing with the extracted juice. We can thus obtain a juice which is free from the poison-saturated fibers.[8]

Even when you are not juicing, eat your fruits and vegetables as close to their raw and natural state as possible. This way, your body can take advantage of the abundant nutrients, enzymes, and fiber provided by them. Our wise Creator has supplied everything needed for our bodies' health within the confines of these natural foods.

Always wash your produce well, even if you purchase organically grown produce. Jay Kordich, (The Juiceman®) who markets the Juiceman® and Juiceman Jr.® machines suggests the following method for removing external contaminants. Mix four tablespoons of salt and the juice of one-half lemon in a sinkful of cold water. Let fruits and vegetables set in it for 5 to 10 minutes. Soak salad (leafy) greens for two to three minutes. Rinse well after soaking. (Note: Some vegetables, such as cucumbers, are frequently waxed. The peels must be removed with a paring knife or peeler.)

It is very important to wash your food, no matter where you buy it. Consider this food for thought: The North

American Free Trade Agreement (NAFTA) was signed into law November 1993. It opened up trade with countries around the world, including Third World countries. This law has been the subject of much controversy. The Public Citizens Global Trade Watch published a comprehensive report on September 24, 1997, regarding food safety as a result of NAFTA. Taking statistics from government, medical, and academic sources, it describes (1) how imported food is more than three times more likely to be contaminated with illegal pesticide residues than U.S.-grown food, (2) while U.S. food imports have skyrocketed, U.S. inspections of imported food have declined significantly, (3) imports of Mexican crops documented by the U.S. government to be at a high risk of pesticide contamination have dramatically increased under NAFTA, (4) foodborne illness is on the rise globally and in the United States, due in part to the "globalization" of the food supply. The contamination is not restricted to pesticides and poisonous sprays. Bacterial contamination originating from body wastes is also a problem, especially with produce from Third World countries. (Note: Some produce will deteriorate quicker if washed and then stored. To retain quality and freshness, wash all commercial produce just before using).

One of them most fascinating books I have ever read about the value of simple foods in restoring health is *The Grape Cure* by Johanna Brandt. First published in the 1920s (no print date is listed), *The Grape Cure* explains how a diet of grapes and grape juice supply all of the necessary materials to help the body overcome cancer and other ailments. Through her personal experience and through those with whom she observed, she learned the power of this single fruit.

It is the only nourishment prescribed in cases of congestion in or adjoining the intestinal tract. After a period of fasting, during which the system is cleansed and prepared for the change of diet, grape juice seems to act as a powerful solvent. At the same time the strength of the patient is maintained by its nourishing properties.

Grapes apparently dissolve the hardened mucus adhering to the walls of the stomach and intestines. In several cases, where the fecal matter was observed, there was an accumulation of stringy, slimy mucus which looked like worms. Sometimes this occurred in long strings, sometimes in clumps resembling balls of string, or sometimes like black and green marbles. The juice appeared to dislodge this accumulation from the walls of the stomach and intestines and act as a flush, carrying it to the rectum. It is therefore considered very important to remove this accumulation by daily enemas, preferably high enemas. When taking only liquids, whether water or fruit juices, daily enemas are deemed necessary, otherwise poisons which have been carried to the intestines by these liquids are likely to be reabsorbed into the blood.

Abnormal growths, cancers, tumors, ulcers, abscesses and fibrous masses seem to be dissolved by the powerful chemical agent in the grape. Diseased tissues and fatty degenerations, every form of morbid matter, is apparently broken up into minute particles and thrown into the blood stream to be carried to the organs of excretion. No wonder then that complications arise. To the inexperienced person it is disconcerting to find strange and new symptoms of disease developing under the "Grape Cure." He needs some-

> one with experience to explain to him that poisons which have been locked up in the system for many years have broken loose and are running riot in the blood. Hence that unusual rise of temperature, that eruption on the skin, those splitting headaches, those attacks of retching and purging, that discharge of mucus, those undue sweatings. The anxious mind of the patient should be set at rest by the assurance that all of these are highly favorable symptoms of the process of purification being carried on internally—positively prove that he is still vital enough to respond to the treatment. The avenues of excretion—the bowels, kidneys, lungs and skin—are still in good working order. Let him then closely examine the stools, the urine, the perspiration, and let him rejoice with the appearance of every new evidence that Nature is still able to cast out the poisons that have been dislodged by the magical action of the grape.[9]

(Author's note: commercial table grapes are among the most toxic and heavily sprayed of all agricultural products. Be absolutely certain that you buy unsprayed grapes from a reliable source. It is interesting to know that when *The Grape Cure* was written, antioxidant compounds known as proanthocyanidins had not been discovered. Today, modern research reveals that grape skin and grape seed extracts are very potent sources of these health-giving antioxidants.)

Milk Is an Imperfect Food

We all grew up being taught that milk is the best source of calcium. It is not. Heavy metals, detergents, antibiotics, viruses, and other toxins have been found in milk. Heavy metals can originate from cows grazing in contaminated areas, and detergent residues can result from the milk machinery cleaning process. Pathogens come from animals that have been weakened and diseased, and then treated to fight their infections. People who are very sensitive to certain antibiotics should be concerned. Residues of drugs are commonly found in milk. Live viral substances have been found in white blood cells of normal and leukemic cattle, as well as in milk, and tissue and cell cultures from the cows.[10]

Milk contains an imbalance of nutrients. It offers a high quantity of sodium and a low quantity of vitamin C and iron. This disparity can contribute to the formation of kidney stones and can also lead to iron deficiency anemia. Calcium and phosphorus are needed to build strong bones and teeth. However, cows' milk contains ten times the amount of calcium and three times as much phosphorus as human milk. This percentage actually causes the calcium to be leached from the bones and can lead to weakening of the bone structure and osteoporosis.[11] High quantities of vitamin D can create a deficiency of magnesium in heart muscle. It is believed that this condition can lead to heart problems in some individuals. Vitamin D is added to commercial milk.[12]

High amounts of xanthine oxidase, an enzyme that is believed to lead to cardiovascular disease, is found in commercial milk. As a result of homogenization, xanthine oxidase is absorbed through the gastrointestinal tract in the fine particles of fat. It proceeds to abrade artery walls and this injury makes it possible for fats to plaque or adhere to the sides of blood vessels.

Synthetic hormones have been used to quickly fatten cattle and are linked to premature puberty in children, especially those who ingest a high amount of animal products. Synthetic hormones are also administered to cows to make them produce more milk. They include BST (bovine somatrophin), also called BGH (bovine growth hormone). The FDA formally approved its use on November 5, 1993.

One cup of carrot juice contains two-and-a-half times more calcium than a comparable glass of milk. It also contains with an abundance of beta carotene, the compound that the body converts to vitamin A. Beta carotene is a superb antioxidant. Antioxidants protect the body from the ravages of toxins, airborne pollutants and many other factors that are known to tear down the immune system, paving the way for cancer and other illnesses. Specifically, beta carotene helps keep mucous membranes healthy. These protective linings are found in the respiratory tract (nose, throat, and lungs) and other areas of the body. Mucous membranes are these tissues' first line of defense against bacteria and viruses. Beta carotene is also essential for healthy eyes, skin and reproduction. The effectiveness of beta carotene will deteriorate rapidly after juicing, so to receive the fullest benefit, it is strongly suggested that you drink your juice immediately after preparation.

What Kind of Juicer Is Best?

There are many juicers on the market today. It would be best to check prices and features on different models before deciding which is best for you. A 1/3 horsepower or 1/2 horsepower juicer would be more expensive than a 1/4 horsepower. However, the 1/4 horsepower model would probably suffice for those not doing an extensive amount of juicing.

Centrifugal juicers operate in a spinning fashion. As it spins and chops at high speeds, the pulp stays inside the basket, separating the juice from the pulp.

Ejector models have two spouts, one on each end. The juice comes out one end, and the pulp the other.

The Champion Juicer is the most popular juicer on the market for overall juicing capabilities. It is known as a "masticator" and beats the fibers, then the juice is strained through a stainless steel mesh. (This process is likened to chewing, hence the nickname). It is a heavy-duty juicer and is good for those who do a lot of juicing.

The hydraulic press juicer, such as the Norwalk juicer, is said to give you 50 to 100 percent more juice containing 3–5 times the vitamins and minerals than juice from other machines. It costs much, much more than the other juicers on the market, but many people who have had chronic illnesses (like cancer) have had great success with the ultimate nutrition this machine provides.

There are special juicers made specifically for extracting the nutrients and chlorophyll in wheatgrass. This juicer is constructed to extract the tiny amount of juice found in the grass. There are both electric and handcrank types on the market.

Preparing for a Juice Fast

Before embarking upon a juice fast for one or two days, your body will have an easier time if you eat only fruits or vegetables for three or four days prior to that time. The transition will be milder and the body will be better prepared to handle the concentrated nutrients supplied in the juices. It is suggested that you drink one to one-and-a-half quarts of juice daily. Some sweet juices like carrot, apple or grape should be diluted half and half with pure distilled water or combined with a "green" juice like celery or kale to avoid stressing the pancreas. Juice fasting will rest the body from the efforts of digestion and assimilation, and will ultimately rejuvenate it. If you employ a fast longer than two days, it is recommended that you do it under the supervision of a health care practitioner (especially if you are under a doctor's care). Babies younger than six months of age shouldn't drink juice. Older babies and young children should be given juices half diluted with water.

Other Sources of Information

There are many excellent books on the market that describe the various juices and their therapeutic uses. One of the most popular is *Raw Vegetable Juices* by Dr. N.W. Walker. First published in 1936, this book pioneered the use of juices to maintain wellness, as well as overcome disease.[13]

There are comprehensive clinical juice programs for serious diseases like cancer and others. They incorporate other natural approaches in addition to juices. A very successful method is employed by The Gerson Institute. It uses the principles of detoxification and rebuilding to heal any disease. Besides cancer, the Institute has successfully treated migraines, psoriasis, chronic fatigue, heart disease, diabetes and a host of other degenerative conditions. The basics of their approach includes drinking 13 glasses daily of various fresh, raw juices prepared hourly from organic fruits and vegetables; eating three complete vegetarian meals made with organic vegetables, fruits and grains; and taking specific nutritional supplements that include pancreatic enzymes. Coffee enemas are used to stimulate the bile ducts to cleanse the liver, so that the liver can cleanse the blood. For more information on this program, call 619-585-7600.

Conclusion

Although not a substitute for a diet that includes fruits and vegetables in their natural state, juicing is the way to get the five or more servings of fruits and vegetables suggested by experts for optimum nutrition. The body needs fiber, as well as vitamins, minerals and enzymes. Juice fasting, on the other hand, can be used periodically to cleanse and rejuvenate the body and release toxins. This can help you feel and look younger, as well as providing abundant energy with which to enjoy life. Start juicing and enjoy health and happiness!

Endnotes

1. Jensen, Bernard, *Foods That Heal*, Garden City Park, New York: Avery Publishing Group, Inc., 1988. 46, 47
2. Santillo, Humbart, *Food Enzymes: The Missing Link to Radiant Health*, Arizona: Hohm Press, 1993. 3,4.
3. Christopher, John R., N.D., M.H., *Dr. Christopher's Natural Healing Newsletter*, Springville: Christopher Publications, Vol. 3, Number 5.
4. Ibid, pp.
5. Wigmore, Dr. Ann. *Dr. Ann Wigmore's Complete Live Food Program*, Massachusetts: Hippocrates Press. 24,60.
6. Walker, Dr. N.W., *Fresh Vegetable and Fruit Juices: What's Missing in Your Body?* Arizona: Norwalk Press, 1970. 82,83.
7. *Mosby's Medical, Nursing, & Allied Health Dictionary*, 3rd Edition, Missouri: The C.V. Mosby Company, 1990. 576.
8. Walker, Dr. N.W,. *Fresh Vegetable and Fruit Juices: What's missing in your body?* Arizona: Norwalk Press, 1970. 17,18.
9. Brandt, Johanna, The Grape Cure, New York: Ehret Literature Publishing Co., Inc. 94-95, 105, 106.
10. "A Multiple Share of Myeloma," *Medical World News*, (May 16, 1969): 23.
11. "Milk Has Something for Everybody?" *JAMA* 232(5), (May 5, 1975): 539.
12. Krause, Marie, *Food, Nutrition, and Diet Therapy*, Philadelphia: W.B. Saunders, 1972. 127.
13. Walker, Dr. N.W., *Raw Vegetable Juices* New York: The Berkeley Publishing Group, 1970.